Screw Infertility!

Screw Infertility!

Lessons from a fertility warrior. Surviving infertility, miscarriage and IVF.

By Robyn Birkin

SCREW INFERTILITY! LESSONS FROM A FERTILITY WARRIOR. SURVIVING INFERTILITY, IVF AND MISCARRIAGE

By Robyn Birkin

Copyright © 2016

ISBN-13: 978-1534610385
ISBN-10: 1534610383

To me, dealing with infertility felt like I'd set off on a 100m sprint, and ended up running a marathon that had no set finish line.

I never knew when it would end, and was constantly searching for strength and stamina in places I never knew existed.

Each time I felt like I couldn't go any further, I discovered that I could, and I did.

There were hurdles, and hills - highs and lows - everywhere.

It was a journey that zapped every last bit of energy from me, like I'd expected to set out on a jog around the block and ended up running miles and miles for my life.

This is the story of my marathon.
My journey of trying to conceive, undergoing fertility treatments, surviving a miscarriage and eventually falling pregnant, with the lessons I want to share with every woman on the heart-wrenching journey through infertility.

For all the fertility warriors out there.

Lessons from a Fertility Warrior

Lesson 1: Sometimes, life just doesn't go to plan

Sometimes you want something so badly, it consumes your entire being. You plan for it, and you expect it to happen for you. But sometimes, no matter how hard you try, no matter how much you plan, how much you deserve it and how much you want it, it's out of reach, and things can come crashing down around you like a tonne of bricks. It just doesn't go to plan.

Like my wedding, which, although it doesn't look like it, was a total disaster. We had eloped to Vanuatu and the wedding was one series of disasters after the next, the pièce de résistance being my husband collapsing at the ceremony with a gastro virus. Night over. After that event I thought that surely I'd used up all my bad luck. That from here on in, all major life events from here on in would be a walk in the park.

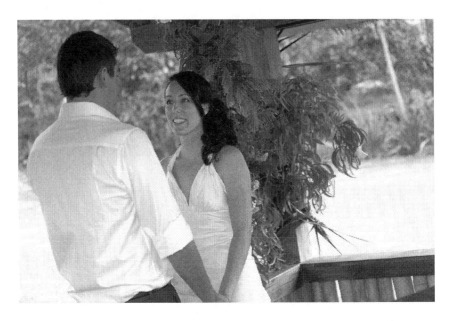

My husband, Rosco and I are high school sweethearts. I still remember the first time I had ever laid eyes on Ross. It was the first day of high school. I had just turned 13 and he had just turned 12. I was in a gaggle of girls as we talked about our previous schools and introduced ourselves. Down the path, a group of boys walked toward us. "That's Ross" said one of my new friends. He had a confident, cheeky smile, long hair tied into a ponytail and was short, like all the boys were at that age as they matured later than the girls. I remember looking into his eyes as he smiled back at me but telling the girls that he wasn't my type.

What I couldn't predict was that we were drawn to each other and that he really was my type: my soul mate. As we made our way through high school, our paths continually crossed, beginning with my first kiss later that year and progressing into a deep friendship and a relationship in our final year of school. We moved out of home when we were 21 and (finally!) got married when we were 28 years old. All around me, my friends were having children, and my boss even used to tell me that she'd hope I wasn't planning any children. Up until the age of 30, I wasn't, and I didn't care that all my friends were having children. At that point, my life was a heady cocktail of working late and attending work functions, date nights, renovating our house and catching up with friends. I was too busy to worry about children. There was plenty of time for that.

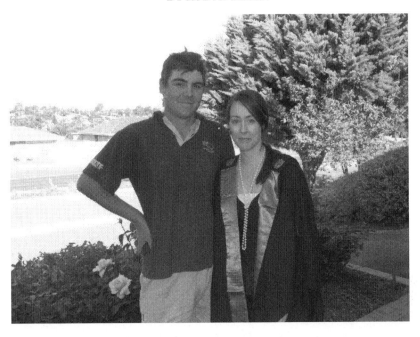

But then I turned 30. And that clock started ticking. And ticking. And ticking. You try to silence that voice in your head that tells you to hurry up. It's impossible to ignore the nagging, but there's also another voice in your head that tells you that so long as you're under 40 you'll be fine.

Was it the right time? Had we done everything we needed to do before having children? Could we afford it? We were full of a million questions and doubts, but we decided (as most people do) that the time would never be perfect, so we plunged forward into preparations to start our family. Making the decision to try for a baby was like an incredible high. We felt a surge of excitement and a renewal of our love as we embarked on this new chapter in our lives together.

I'd done did everything right on a woman's 'timeline of life'. Find a man, check. Get married, check. Buy a house together, check. Travel the world, check. Build a high flying career, check.

Having a child was next on the list. This was the next logical step and it was the right time.

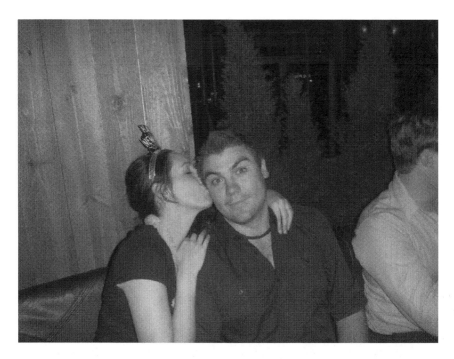

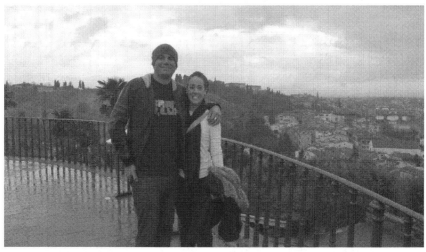

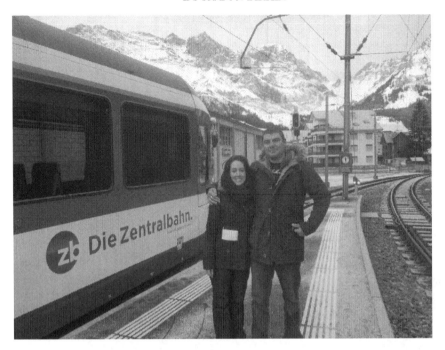

I'd seen naturopaths before and had never really clicked. This chick seemed like the real deal. She was gorgeous and slim with long, shiny, blonde hair, a bounce in her step and looked like she lived what she preached. All I could think was 'I want what she's having!' My last naturopath had greasy skin, pimples, and a muffin top, and was constantly trying to fleece my wallet, putting me on a diet that involved 101 powders, potions and protein bars that she, of course, sold. Every time I left her office I felt used and deflated.

But I felt a connection with this new naturopath. On my first consultation, I lay on the massage table and relaxed as she tapped and prodded my arms, legs, head and wrists. Part of me wanted to laugh at how ridiculous this must seem from the outside, but I relaxed in the knowledge that this was the first time all week I'd had to just sit still. Leaving her office I felt a little woozy. A little relaxed. And happy. I'd had sleep issues for years and after that first night, I slept like a baby. And then I woke feeling refreshed and recharged. When I'd arrive at her office each week, she'd ask "How are you feeling?" and I always felt like this was an hour that was dedicated to me. I could truly reply with the way my body was physically feeling and how I was feeling emotionally. And I could just lay there, without having to worry about what I was cooking for dinner, or the next deadline at work. It was me time. It was therapy.

It turns out that she specialised in fertility. How convenient. And then we started her fertility plan: three months of detoxing and preparing your body for pregnancy. This was all part of my grand plan. I was sold. And in true Capricorn fashion, I'd planned and prepared for success. Getting pregnant would be a walk in the park, I assured myself.

We leapt forward into the pre-conception plan. I was taking supplements, including pre-natal vitamins, and herbs, and embarked on an elimination diet, saw me give up gluten, soy, alcohol and basically all other pleasures in life! I was on a mission, and dedicated to the task.

I had recently become vegetarian too and, as part of this diet I was meant to be giving up dairy but just the thought of giving up dairy seemed impossible. If I gave up dairy too there'd be nothing in the world for me to eat other than lettuce, rice and beans! So the dairy stayed, but everything else was kicked to the curb in the name of supercharging my body for pregnancy success. I was exercising four times a week, and I was oh so confident that this would be a walk in the park. I was incredibly excited. I was doing everything right and I felt physically great.

I remember one day, two months into the three month plan saying to Ross, "do you really actually think we're ready? Maybe we should hold off a little while longer? Naaahhh." We were supposed to try and use protection during that time and we were pretty good, but also pretty carefree at the same time, just using loose protection methods like the 'pull out method' and secretly giggling to ourselves behind my naturopath's back that we just could actually fall pregnant before we were even trying. It felt like a naughty secret. She gave me a tracking chart and explained to me how to track my cycle. Each morning I'd lay still and studiously track my temperature, cervical mucous and became hyper aware of my moods, trying to look for any pattern I could. This was how the manic mindset of fertility began. It began with once a day noting where I was on my cycle and just that act alone, meant that I knew roughly what time of month was the optimal time to conceive and once you know that piece of information, you spend the first half of the month eagerly waiting for that moment of ovulation, and the next part of the month anticipating the result. Every moment of the day was spent analysing symptoms of either ovulation or pregnancy. Day 1, Day 2, Day 3......

Finally, the third month was over, and we were ready to try. We were jumping out of our pants with excitement. It was happening right now. We were going to become parents and embark on this exciting journey together.

NOBODY knew we were trying. My parents had no grandchildren, and were itching to become grandparents. One day my dad blurted out, "You know, if you couldn't have children, you would just adopt." What the? On the outside I was like 'Pffftttt....left field. Whatever.' Inside I was like 'little do you know that soon we'll be pregnant! Mu ha ha ha.'

It was right around the time that the book, *50 Shades of Grey* came out, and while we didn't create a red room or invest in any whips, the thought of finally making love to try and have a baby and the release of this novel that celebrated an active sex life was an exhilarating high! I visited the adult shop and purchased raunchy underwear and made sure we invested the time into enjoying the process. It felt so naughty, yet so purposeful. Life was great and I was pumped to be starting this new chapter in our lives. We did everything by the books that first month, and I imagined how beautiful the experience would be, and how we would recall 'that weekend' when we conceived our son or daughter. Then came the wait, which was exciting but also went really slowly. Two weeks felt like two years. All I could think was 'I wonder if I'm pregnant?' and 'I could be pregnant right now.' I looked up how long it would take for us to know and saw that it could tell us within seven days. I was just dying to know if we were pregnant and couldn't help but take myself to the store to buy a pregnancy test. The anticipation grew as I took the test, confident that I would soon see two red lines… but it was negative. Huh. And then I googled the symptoms of pregnancy and started analysing every hiccup and sensation in my body, wondering whether it was a sign that I was expecting. I waited a few days and bought another test. Negative. Huh. Finally my period came (which was unmistakable for an implantation bleed) and I remember feeling this huge sense of confusion and disappointment. I felt like I had nailed the preparation for this and it didn't happen for me. It was like building a rocket and preparing for take-off and the bloody thing won't ignite. But, not everyone falls pregnant straight away, so that was fine, I told myself. It was totally normal to not conceive in the first month, and I continued on, still expecting it to happen each month.

When I went to see my naturopath she said that everything looked fine and to keep trying. There was nothing in our way. She looked at my charts and we discussed when we thought I was ovulating. Things were still exciting in the bed, but it was starting to feel like Groundhog Day. It was no longer like I was getting frisky in the bed with the bonus of falling pregnant. It was more like a military plan: I would track my basal body temperature each morning and know exactly when I was ovulating, and then we would make love as much as we could during that time, and when we did, I would lay there on the bed for 20 minutes with my hips and legs elevated to try and increase our chances of conceiving… while I Googled whether doing that actually did increase the chances.

But each month, I would discover I wasn't pregnant. And each month sex would become a little less enjoyable and a little more forced. And each month of trying hopelessly, another small part of me died. I went to a friend's 30th birthday and she started crying because she wanted to have a third child and her husband was happy with two. Inside I just kept thinking that I'd be happy with just one. I WISHED I'd had her problem. I listened to her as she sobbed, telling us about how she would write a letter to her husband telling him how much she wanted a child, but glazing over the details as my mind was consumed by my own thoughts of wanting, longing for a child. I was surrounded by my best friends, but couldn't tell them about our struggle. I desperately wanted to pour my heart out to them and reveal my pain... our pain... but then the cat would be out of the bag. I had to maintain my poker face and a smile. This had become the story of my life.

A friend in my team at work fell pregnant. I remember sitting in the lunchroom, quietly dying inside, while she told us all how her Doctor remarked that she must be SO fertile, because she had fallen pregnant after a crazy night on the booze, just a few days after she had gone off the pill. I watched her incredibly gorgeous belly growing, the glow on her face, and her incredible happiness, month after month, while wrestling with my own ambivalence. I was thrilled for her. So glad for her, and I enjoyed seeing her blossom, while unable to stop comparing myself to her, and the reminder that each month and week further along she became in her pregnancy, was months and weeks that we were still trying without success. The distance between us kept growing.

Then, I went to breakfast with a friend who told me she was expecting her third child, and all I could think was that if I'd fallen pregnant, I'd be having a baby at the same time too, and my heart sank yet again. All of a sudden, it felt like everyone was pregnant except me. Even Kate Middleton was pregnant! Aarrrgghhh. My world felt like it was slowly shrinking and I gradually felt more isolated. And desperate. Why wasn't this happening for us? How long would it take? I just wanted the answer. Wasn't there a higher power that could just tell me when this would all end? When would we ever fall pregnant, so this awful, agonising suspense would end? Here was my friend, having her third child, and I couldn't even bear one. I felt like I was falling behind and could never catch up, but once again I feigned happiness and a straight face and continued on. I casually quizzed her on the details: how long it had taken her to fall pregnant (first cycle... gahhh) and how she'd tracked it. She said she had bought ovulation and pregnancy kits from Ebay. Oh my. That opened a door and added fuel to my fire of desperation. That night I went online and purchased a bulk pack of these kits, and the obsession started to take hold. Peeing on a stick was much easier than sitting there every morning with a thermometer in my mouth, laying as still as I could and clamping my mouth shut for 10 minutes, trying to test my temperature to see when I was ovulating, and the little sticks for testing were so cheap. I burned through those sticks. My naturopath didn't have any answers for me - I was healthy! Six months of trying, and by this stage, I was a complete mess.

It was all I'd think about, day and night. I almost felt like I could hear the seconds hand clock at every moment, as life ticked by ever so slowly. How could I think of anything else? I was painfully aware at each moment of the day and month of what stage of my cycle I was in and how much of a failure we'd been until now. I would be obsessed with when we should have sex. It had become robotic and mechanical. My libido was nonexistent. Sex was a necessary chore. I almost dreaded it because of the failure I was expecting at the end of the month. It was just another reminder of what I was supposed to be doing, my duty in life as a women, and what I couldn't do. My one job on earth at a basic, primal level was to have children, and I couldn't. There was no biological point to my being on earth. Yet each month, I'd have a desperate slither of hope and expectation that it would work. I'd analyse every faint symptom of pregnancy and count down the hours and days until there was the possibility of a positive pregnancy test. And then I would test, each day until I got my period. I was so desperate and delusional that when I started to get my period I'd always try and convince myself that it was an embryo implanting, a sign of pregnancy and that perhaps the bleeding would stop soon and I'd be pregnant. And when the bleeding didn't stop and I finally realised that there was no possible way I was pregnant, I'd be a crying mess on the floor of the bathroom. I would just sit there and cry and cry, wishing that I could stop time, find the answer as to what was wrong or when this would finally work, or just take my mind off infertility for just a moment. It was all consuming. I'd been working on this for nine months, and only my husband and naturopath knew. I just felt utterly alone.

What was the problem? I prayed, constantly, that I could just find the answers - the why, the how, the when! Oh, the when. There was nothing else we could do though aside from just keep trying.

I gave up exercising as a last ditch effort, thinking that I would just treat my body gently at every step. Maybe that was it?

Maybe I was exercising too much. Maybe it really was dairy? So, that was it. I gave up dairy, and once again ditched gluten. I gave up coffee, alcohol, soy – everything on the elimination list again. Maybe it was Ross. He needs to go see the naturopath too! We did everything. If someone had told me that in order to fall pregnant, I needed to spend at least 30 minutes a day, hopping on one foot, singing Old MacDonald and that would increase our chances of falling pregnant, I'd have done it.

Months passed again. The desperation grew. So did the panic and sadness. And the pregnant people around me. And the first birthday parties. What was, in reality, 12 months of waiting, until we had passed that period of waiting until we could finally visit our GP and get an appointment at a Fertility Clinic, felt like a lifetime. We finally had our Doctor appointment, an admission that it wasn't working. "It's so hard," I said as I burst into tears in her office. I couldn't even control myself anymore.

Finally, the day had arrived for us to see a specialist about our situation. Of all days, it was on Valentine's Day. We arrived at the fertility clinic for our appointment and were referred for a huge number of tests - blood tests, physical tests, internal tests. Finally though, I felt like it was kind of out of our hands. We'd find out what was wrong and move on. And it was like we had acceptance that something really wasn't right and someone was going to take charge and fix it. There was a huge part of me that was reluctant to trust our specialist though. Years of seeing uncaring general practitioners had left me cynical and untrusting of the medical industry. I didn't want to take drugs and ruin all the good I had spent years cultivating in my body. I was HEALTHY goddamit. I was into wellness and green smoothies, dammit. There must have just been a glitch in the matrix somewhere. I couldn't understand why this was happening to me, to us. We didn't deserve this.

The specialist split Ross and I into separate rooms and I was told to debrief and lay on the bench while the Doctor did a quick examination, methodically and robotically, as if he had done it 1000 times before. I could feel my dignity slowly sinking to the floor. I could foresee months of opening my legs for complete strangers in my future. Ross was handled in much the same manner.

While we were waiting on our results and our next appointment with our specialist, we'd do a month of blood tests to check my hormone levels during the month and check if my hormones were doing what they were supposed to, and also let us know when to have the hanky panky in case we were just off with our timing. My results were perfect. Textbook even.

I arrived at the radiological clinic for yet another test. I was told it would be painful, and given some painkillers to take beforehand. I arrived and was taken to a cubicle where I undressed and changed into just a hospital gown, and then made my way down the corridor to where a group of people waited, to check if I had blocked tubes, just one more procedure to rule out on this journey of discovery. I laid on the cold, metal bed with my legs akimbo, while they put the dye up there as I tried hard to look anywhere but in anyone's eyes. It felt almost humiliating, and embarrassing but I tried to focus all my energy on appearing calm and composed. I tried to fixate on a point on the ceiling. Physically, it felt fine. And then all of a sudden I felt the most awful cramp that grew suddenly like a tsunami. It was utterly horrible. It was agony. 10 out of 10. I wanted to double up in pain. I wanted out. I wanted to crawl up in a burl and roll around on the floor. Now! But I had to lay still. I didn't know how much I could take. "Stay still," the lady kept saying while I lay there, desperately trying to focus and stay still while my body was screaming at me to move. I started taking deep breaths, holding in the tears while my eyes felt like they were about to burn a hole in the ceiling of the room as I tried to focus… and then, in an instant it was over. I was given a large pad thing and told to walk back to the toilets and change room holding it. They had curtained off the hallway to the toilets so nobody could go past while I walked there and I know why. The liquid just kept pouring out of me like I'd wet my pants, yet another one of the series of dignity defying acts I would undertake on this journey through hell.

So then the moment of truth when we got our test results back. Turns out my husband is missing some chromosomes. How do people just 'miss' chromosomes? I thought. We were referred to genetic counsellors. We were given the number by our clinic to call them. That week, I dialled the number. "You can't just call us," said the lady on the other end of the line. "But, but, my fertility clinic gave me your number and told me to call," I replied, confused. "No, you need to be referred to us, you can't just call us," she said. I was confused. We had been referred. This is what I was trying to tell her. Our fertility clinic had found an abnormality and had given us the referral and told us to make an appointment? As I explained this to her, she still didn't seem to understand. "The fertility clinic HAS referred us. My husband is missing some chromosomes. They've sent you a referral and I have a printed copy too," I said. I could feel her frustration at me, but I was doing what my clinic had told me to do and this was our lives. I couldn't decipher these results on my own and we needed to know what impact this had on our fertility. "Well, we'll wait until we receive your clinic's referral and then we'll call you," she bluntly announced. I was bemused at how a counsellor could be so insensitive, when surely they're dealing daily with people who have just been told potentially life-altering news, but I left it at that. A few weeks later they called Ross at work. "We've received your referral and we don't believe this has an impact on your fertility. Is this phone call enough or do you feel that you need to come in?" the lady advised. "Umm, no this phone call is fine?" said Ross.

While we were glad that this supposedly didn't have any impact on his fertility, and glad we no longer had to deal with the negative energy of the genetic counselling clinic, we were left confused. Since when do we have chromosomes in our body that do nothing? Was it just that science didn't yet know what these chromosomes did? What else would our tests uncover?

Everything else was kind of ok. I never expected that. I was expecting them to find a big, red, flashing sign that pointed to our problem, but there wasn't. His tests were kind of ok - nothing special, on the low side of normal, but no red flags. It was a bit of a letdown to be honest. And this is how our fertility treatments began - the blood tests, the drugs, the fertility treatments, while Ross was retested. We were ushered into a room with a nurse as we were bombarded with information about what we needed to do, and a calendar of how the month would progress, and given a tutorial on how to inject myself, leaving with a haul of drugs and paperwork in my hands and my mind spewing with instructions and details of what we needed to do next. There was a part of me that thought this was all a joke. Injecting myself? Oh my, how hardcore I thought I was. Sticking pessaries up my bottom? How hilarious. And I thought that I was dealing with it all really well. This was serious, and I needed to laugh to get through it. Otherwise, I'd cry. Well actually, I cried too. One thing's for sure though. Things definitely weren't going to plan.

I remember the first time I injected myself. As I tried to carefully measure the dosage and steady my arm, it almost seemed impossible to punch the needle through my skin. It wasn't only the physical act of injecting myself so much as the comparison I felt to a junkie who was reliant on a needle to get by, or a diabetic who much in the same way needed to inject themselves daily. Never in a million years did I think I'd have a sharps disposal container by my bedside, sitting on the edge of my bed, trying to summon the courage to medicate myself, and finally coming to terms with the fact that if we were ever to have a child, it would not be in the traditional sense like everyone else, it would be at the hands of science. I was one of the statistics now. We had infertility.

Lesson 2: Stop suffering in silence

Once we had come to accept that having a child naturally was not an option for us, the time had come. We couldn't hold this secret in any longer and so we told our parents who were amazingly supportive, although full of a million questions. It felt like a small weight had been lifted off our shoulders. We gradually told the rest of our family too. I felt like I had been carrying this burden of sadness for such a long time all on my own. This feeling of utter failure, of desperation and always trying to keep a brave, poker face, not being able to share these feelings with anyone else, took every ounce of energy I had, like my ship had capsized and I was left there, alone, treading water with sharks circling around me.

I went away for the weekend with my girlfriends, my tribe. All weekend I'd wanted to tell them about our struggle but the time just wasn't right. At dinner, drinking on the balcony, sitting in our pyjamas chatting at night. So many moments passed when I had wanted to tell them, but couldn't quite summon the courage, and then all of a sudden at breakfast, I burst into tears and blurted out that we were having fertility treatments. I couldn't even look them in the eyes as I described our journey to four women who all had children and couldn't truly comprehend my pain. At first they just sat there looking at me like stunned mullets, not quite knowing what to say, or perhaps still digesting the words they hadn't expected to hear that morning. As I continued telling our story, I could feel their pain for me, and they began to open up and ask questions.

But, each time we told someone it got easier and easier. There were a million questions, but it was like all of a sudden, the conversation shifted from 'when are you going to have kids?' to 'what happens next?' and other questions about fertility treatments and I could focus on explaining treatments and the process, rather than having my own pity party and wallowing in my pain on my own.

Seeing my naturopath was my sanctuary. Once a month, I had the chance to sit down, relax, and have someone ask (and genuinely want to know) how I was going. It was like therapy. Here was someone who had an hour of my time, just to focus on ME and how I was feeling, both inside and out, and help me work through ways to cope. I'd lay on her massage table while she did her thing, as she told me stories about herself and asked me questions. It was a moment to relax and not feel like I had to keep a brave face.

The ovulation inductions didn't work. My body produced too many eggs the first time around so the first one was cancelled, and the second one didn't work either. And then Ross's tests came back fine, which left us really in the dark. There really was no smoking gun. We then had two cycles of Intrauterine Insemination. By this stage, I thought I was getting through pretty well. By this stage, everyone knew. All of our friends and family, and even my work, who were really supportive. It was much easier now that everyone knew, and I didn't have too many side effects from the medications. I felt lighter and not as burdened by this great weight on my shoulders. I thought I was coasting through this, although it all still takes longer than you ever imagine. It takes longer to get appointments, longer to get test results and then meet to your specialist, and when one cycle fails, time to reset for the next. It all takes time. Much longer than you initially expect.

I'd had four months off dairy, and actually felt great. I'd dropped at least five kilograms without even trying, but then one night I went out with Ross for a meal and decided that I'd start eating dairy again. Big mistake. I had the worst stomach cramps. Turns out that dairy really doesn't agree with me, so dairy free meals were here to stay. In the space of a year, I'd overhauled my diet completely, and I had also absorbed and inhaled every article I could about toxic chemicals in everyday products my lifestyle had changed completely. I was changing as a person too. My mission to become pregnant had taken over my entire life.

Lesson 3: Do what you can manage

I was determined though to make this happen, so I started seeing an acupuncturist. Oh my, that was awkward. I'd sit there embarrassingly talking about my breast fullness, my bowel movements and my cycles to a 30-something Chinese man. Oh man! And then, when I got up on the massage bench, he took my bra straps off to put needles in. I lay there wondering if this was possibly the most awkward, cringe worthy moment of my life. At times he wanted to see me several times per week, and it was exhausting. I'd lay there during treatments and some days there was music, other days there was silence, but my mind would race the entire time. I was wired and consumed with trying to fall pregnant and it was different to my naturopath's office - I just couldn't relax there. I was taking his supplements, plus supplements from my naturopath, plus a tonne of other random things like fertility bracelets for good luck, and money was flying out of my wallet faster than it was coming in. It was too much.

Every second question I had from people was what the next step in treatment was, and when we'd have our next result. I felt much less alone now that everyone knew, but it almost felt like we had no privacy anymore. And it still hurt when people announced their pregnancies, or had babies or invited me to their children's parties. I wasn't angry at them or resentful, so much as it reminded me of what I didn't have and desperately wanted. It was just sadness. And tiredness. Like I had been running a marathon on a treadmill.

The year before we'd began trying for a baby I was at the baby shower of a close friend, and she had another friend there, Annette. There were only three of us there who didn't have children. One was me (who secretly in the back of my head had an inkling that we'd begin trying at 30), another friend who was single, and Annette. I have clear vision of her saying "Oh yuck. Kids, no. Nowhere near that point." And then one day at the supermarket I ran into her. And she was about eight months pregnant. My heart just sank, like the anchor of a ship dropping to the bottom if the ocean and crashing on the ocean floor. Of all the people in the world, and even though I didn't know her that well, I think there was a part of me that thought that although everyone else around me was having children, at least she wasn't there yet. And then she was. I just panicked. She was having a baby too, just like everyone else. At that moment it felt like I was the only person in the world who didn't have a child. I was truly alone. I had to get out of there. I could feel myself start to hyperventilate and my world started crashing down around me and I just blurted out "hi, oh congratulations, gotta run, sorry I'm running late for something," and I turned, and walked straight out, trying to breathe and hold my tears in until I at least made it to the car. I raced home, walked through the front door and straight onto our bed, bursting into tears. This was awful. We were supposed to have children before her, and we were getting left behind. Ross heard me sobbing and came to the bedroom, and looked at me, confused and unsure of what he was supposed to do. I cried all the time, and so frequently that he felt helpless, and useless at comforting me.

This wasn't natural selection at all. We were healthy, middle class, mentally stable people. We would make incredible parents. Meanwhile, all these people, like drug addicts and child abusers, who shouldn't, are popping out children. This was unfair. Where was Mother Nature? She was getting it all wrong. And then there were stories of people who stopped trying and then miraculously fell pregnant. Someone's husbands, friends, sisters, cousin, no doubt.

"And why didn't we just adopt?"
"Or had we tried just going on a holiday?"
"And we should really just try to stop stressing?"
EVERYONE NEEDED TO SHUT UP!!!

The acupuncturist wanted to see me weekly and a times, bi-weekly. Combined with the sometimes daily hospital blood tests, trying to do gentle walking, my newfound crazy diet, seeing my naturopath and working crazy hours, I just felt frazzled. So much for trying to stop stressing. I was determined to fall pregnant but it's hard not to let the obsession take over. I was militant about what I ate. I gave up coffee and alcohol. I didn't eat any junk food. It was too much.

Almost every second of every day consumed me with our fertility. When you have a cycle at a clinic and they monitor your bloods you need to be at clinic at a certain time of the morning. And the rooms are full. You're desperately trying to cling to any elements of your life that resemble normalcy, like your job, that begins at 8.00am, but they only open for bloods at 7.00am and you get there at 6.30am and write your name on the list and then wait. And wait. And wait. And wait for your name to be called. If you get there at 7.00am, you'll be much farther down the queue and be late, yet again, for work. For some of us, the half an hour before the clinic opens is spent sitting in the car park, because the clinic won't open the doors until a particular time. We listen to the radio or read a book, consumed by our problems, and surrounded by women just like us in a packed fertility clinic, yet never feeling so as isolated as we do in those moments. And then we need to make sure we are available at a particular time that day to take our test results and find out the next step that and afternoon. We spend all day watching the clock and pondering our fate until we make or take that call. When we are waiting on a pregnancy result, the wait is agonising.

I gave up the acupuncture. I'd been trying it for four months and I still hadn't fallen pregnant, and I felt I had given it a fair shot. I had to do what I could to manage. It was like I had a dinner plate. The fertility treatment was my meat, my friends and family were my potatoes, and my lifestyle was my veggies. There was only so much of everything I could fit on my plate, so I needed to stick to a balance that worked for me emotionally. Just cutting out that one activity to free up my schedule and my mind made a huge difference to the way I was feeling. I felt like I could breathe again.

We had yet another appointment with our fertility specialist. It was time to bring out the big guns: IVF. There was a part of me that had been hoping the whole time that we'd just move to IVF and get the show on the road. I was done waiting! The specialist explained the process to us and talked about how they extract the eggs - by basically punching a hole in your uterus and sucking them out. And how they would most likely only ever put one egg back in…. And he told me some stuff about how the risks are increased with twins and triplets and blah blah blah blah, because I tuned out because inside I was just thinking 'OMG I'd LOVE twins! Then I could get this all done in one shot! Please, please, please can we somehow miraculously have twins,' I thought as visions of myself holding two babies at the same time dizzily swirled through my mind.

Lesson 4: Even though sometimes you feel alone, you aren't.

As part of starting IVF, we were required to sign a tonne of paperwork, attend an information session, and also see a counsellor. The paperwork was in-depth. We had to think of scenarios like what we would do with fertilised eggs if we decided we didn't want anymore kids, and Ross had to give his permission for me to use his sperm if, in-between treatment he suddenly died. We had never even considered any of this! And, if we had eggs we didn't want to use anymore, would we dispose of them, donate them to science or possibly donate them to another couple? Although if we donated them to another couple, it was a little bit like adoption in that the kids could still contact us. It was heavy stuff. And things that are really hard to decide until you're in that moment.

And then there were those other two things. The information session and the mandatory counselling session. I couldn't help but think they would have been helpful at the start of our journey and I still do. When you first begin seeing a fertility clinic, you've already been through months and months of heartache, and don't really have any idea what the process is or what the success rates of the clinic are or how they like to operate. You have no idea really what ovulation induction is or what the different types of medication are. By the time you get to IVF, you're an expert! You've spent enough hours googling things to earn a degree in…. well… googling. And you've already had to spend nearly every waking hour learning how to deal with your infertility.

But they were compulsory, so we attended them. There were a few golden nuggets in the information session. Mostly I was just blown away by how many other people were there. The room was full. Here we are in today's society, with one in six couples suffering with infertility, and undergoing fertility treatments, but we are like a silent sorority. And now we were crammed into a room together to watch a powerpoint presentation from a lab technician and a clinic manager.

And the counselling session. What a waste of time. The lady was about 65 years old, and had never gone through the emotional rollercoaster of infertility herself. She gave us some cookie cutter advice like 'stay busy.' It wasn't totally useless, and I'm sure there are many people who may benefit from it, but, one of the reasons I'm now so passionate about helping women survive infertility is because of my experience and feeling like there was not a lot out there to help us get through this massive experience emotionally. I wanted to speak with other people in the same situation as me. I wanted to speak with fertility warriors and hear their stories and be comforted by others who had gone through what I'd been through and survived. I wanted desperately to know that everything would be ok. I wanted to engage with other people who knew how I felt! Where was that connection? So I started to build my own community, my own group of warriors who were going through the same journey as me. And ticked those three boxes so we could get the show on the road.

Our first ever IVF cycle began just like the rest of them, but finished in a way that would change my life forever. As per usual, the drugs went gangbusters in my body. I was always on the minimum dose of everything, yet still my body would freak out and produce a large number of eggs. When I had my ultrasound, they counted 39 growing eggs inside my ovaries. I could even feel my belly bulging a bit and the pressure on my stomach when I sat down. Finally, the time had come to get this show on the road - I was going to have IVF and this was going to happen. I arrived at the hospital, ready for what was about to begin and was escorted up to my private hospital room. It all felt very glamorous and a little bit exciting, as my sadness was momentarily distracted by the fancy hospital room and excitement at this progressive next step. I met with the anaesthetist who cracked some jokes and asked me some questions, and then I was wheeled into a sterile room for surgery, where the fertility specialist sat glued to his computer, not even stopping to say hello and the lab technician stood, ready for his part in this science experiment. The anaesthetist and his assistant cracked jokes and made me feel like a human being, probably trying to distract me from all the needles they were placing in my arms and the mask they were putting over my face. Just before they put me under, the lab technician blurted out that there might be a chance my implantation would be cancelled because of my risk of complications from the treatment, a rare side effect called Ovarian Hyperstimulation Syndrome. "Sorry whaaaa……?" Too late, I was under. Only 3% of women get it. I wasn't worried. Whatever. Waking up in the hospital, I was greeted by a nurse who said that she had two twins via IVF. "How many eggs did they get?" I asked, wondering how many rolls of the dice I would get. "They got 15 eggs," she replied. Part of me was a little confused because there were so many eggs on my scans. More than 15! I was also proud of myself for being such a fantastic egg-making machine. But I was groggy. 'How many eggs did she say again?' I wondered as I was still consumed by the fog of anesthesia. I knew that I had just asked her, but suddenly could not recall at all how many eggs she said they'd retrieved. I asked again and she replied. Like Groundhog Day, I then asked again. It was like I had no short term memory. After going around in circles for about 30 minutes with a very kind and patient nurse, I was wheeled back to my bedroom. When I arrived back, it was time for lunch. I had ordered the vegan option. I had written about my meal preference on multiple forms - my pre-admission form, when the nurse asked me before going into surgery, yet here I was being served fish. I couldn't eat that. Didn't they know that I'd overhauled my lifestyle and fish was no longer part of it? I apologised to the nurse and said I couldn't eat it, but she explained that until I had eaten something they wouldn't discharge me, so she took the meal back and called the kitchen. They brought me a vegetarian meal and I felt like such an inconvenience, but I told the nurse again that I couldn't eat it. Once again she called the kitchen, and I could overhear her saying "Yep, no dairy or eggs,. No dairy and eggs. She is vegan" and before long my third meal arrived. It was fish again. What the hell? By this time, even the nurse was dismayed and I told her I'd just drink the apple juice and then get my dad to guarantee he'd buy me something to eat on my way back home. She'd gone from insistent to defeated and agreed. Following the surgery I felt pretty good but rested for the remainder of the day, inhaling a vegan burrito, after being picked up from my 'hotel room' by my dad.

The following day we eagerly awaited a phone call, wondering when the suspense would end. Finally they called and told us that only three eggs had fertilised. What a disappointment. Those were crap figures. My heart sank. I had just assumed that nearly all of them would fertilise. Was I naive? We were told they were all top grade eggs though and that was something, but the lab technician said that I should have had 75% of my eggs fertilise, not the result I had. It was yet another low on this journey, although I tried to remain positive with what I had. After all, I knew people who had only extracted one egg before!

48 hours later we were back in the clinic. By this time I was really quite bloated, but I kept downing my water and gatorade as they'd requested, and going to the toilet every five seconds too. In truth, I had tried anything I could to not have to drink the gatorade because I was trying to be so health conscious. I had bought coconut water, but for some reason it tasted foul. I had added Himalayan salt to my water, but there was only so much I could drink, and when I ran out of options, I surrendered and ended up just drinking the goddam gatorade. Because of my risk of this complication called OHSS, I had to get there an hour early for an

assessment to see if it would go ahead or not. I was feeling pumped and excited though. This was our chance! The nurse measured my abdominal width and weighed me and asked me a tonne of questions about how I was feeling, and then I was ushered back into the waiting room, while they had a little whisper to the Doctor as they decided whether or not to let us go ahead, as I desperately wished that everyone in the waiting room would be quiet and the phone would stop ringing so I could hear what they were saying.

They came out and the Doctor sat with us and asked us what we wanted to do. Of course we said "go ahead." Have they ever had someone who hasn't said yes? I didn't care about much other than falling pregnant as soon as humanly possible. So what if I had a bit of bloating? I was just desperate for this heartache to be over, and I didn't care what it took. This gut-wrenching marathon seemed to never end. I was tired. Exhausted. Of course I was going to say yes! They went ahead with the egg they thought had the best chance of success, although none of them had really multiplied much. What did that mean? I didn't know, but we forged ahead. As they placed the egg in my uterus I could see my little embryo shoot out of the tube with a little puff like a shooting star. In a twisted way it was kind of romantic. Just like that it was over, and yet another two week wait was ahead of us.

Less than a week later though I could barely walk or breathe. I sounded like I was constantly out of breath. I was sleeping in the spare room sat upright with pillows all around me because I was so uncomfortable. It was torture. I had accumulated seven kilograms of fluid in my abdomen. It had taken up all the space in my belly and the skin had stretched so much I was walking hunched over like the hunchback of Notre Dame, and the skin was firm and tight. It hadn't had time to stretch and my body didn't have time to adjust from this massive influx of fluid. You know that feeling when you're hungover and you just feel like if you even just roll over in the bed, you'll throw up? That's how I felt. And I looked like I was five months pregnant –the irony was incredible.

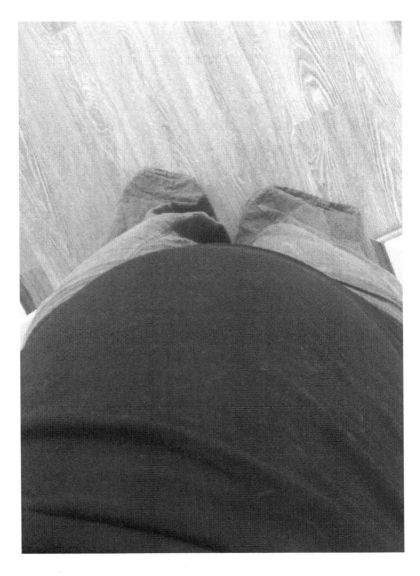

I needed to go in on New Year's Eve for a blood test and I struggled. The appointments are early in the morning, I just felt incredibly nauseous, weak and horrible - going into the clinic was the last thing I felt like doing. But I did because I had no choice. I shuffled, hunched over with one hand on my stomach and the other clutching a water bottle, and just went straight to the reception desk and groaned "I need to see a nurse." They knew something wasn't right and suddenly, the clinic jolted into action. This was their most undesired side effect of treatment. I was rushed in to see the nurse who examined me and then called one of the specialists. He hastily organised an ultrasound to assess the damage. My stomach was at the top of my chest where my lungs were, my bowels pushed toward my spine, as my organs fought for space in this cramped space amongst seven kilograms of floating fluid in my abdomen. Yet despite the abundance of liquid in my body, I was incredibly dehydrated. I was downing all of this water and gatorade but it was just spewing out of my body and into the abyss, instead of nourishing me. They considered whether to admit me into hospital, but I didn't see the point when I could essentially just keep drinking water. In the time that had passed since the transfer I had spent many wakeful hours scouring the internet for the experiences of others who had suffered with ovarian hyperstimulation syndrome and I knew that I didn't want to be admitted, but I felt like death and I just wanted to badly to be able to take a deep breath and stand up straight. It was now a moderate case of OHSS. My progesterone levels were through the roof. 20 times more than what they should be. My body had once again gone gangbusters on the medication, which explained the extreme nausea I was feeling.

The good news though, was that I was pregnant. Finally. All of this time, I had been waiting for this miracle, and now I just had to focus on getting well again and I'd be able to enjoy this little person growing inside me. I tried to focus on the happiness of achieving this goal rather than the discomfort and pain I was in.

Lesson 5: Control what you tell people. This is your journey.

The relief was overwhelming. I finally felt like I could survive the hyperstimulation and that it was all part of a bigger plan. The immediate pain and discomfort I was feeling became somewhat bearable, and I felt like I could see the finish line of this marathon. I'd lay there, rubbing my swollen buddha tummy, reflecting on this journey and how brave I was. Of course, everyone was asking whether I was pregnant, because they all knew about the IVF cycle. Of course they did, because they asked and I had told them. The moment you finally tell people about your situation, not only do they become experts, and seem to know someone who took a holiday and a break from trying and miraculously fell pregnant naturally, but they also think they have the right to ask you about every intimate step in the process, including on what day you'll find out if you're pregnant. And on that day, you are overwhelmed by curious souls wanting to know the outcome. They do it because they love you. They do it because they care. But in that moment, you just want to be around people who understand the treatments and outcomes, and now that you're pregnant, you just want to feel like a normal person instead of a science experiment again, and normal people have the luxury and excitement of this little secret. This little bubble of happiness that they get to share with people at the 12 week mark once they have their first proper scan.

We told our parents, but that was all and were just a bit cagey with everyone else. "Oh, they're just doing some further tests on things," I'd answer. I knew I was pregnant. Let's be honest, they probably did too.

From that moment on, I was glad I had told people about our journey, but knew that from now I had to control just what information I gave, despite what questions they asked. I had discovered that my role didn't need to be of teacher to them, and that just because we were going through fertility treatments and made that open, it didn't mean that they needed to know every detail. And it was ok for me to tell people when I didn't want to discuss things anymore. I just needed to be straight up and honest and not mince my words.

The ritual of blood tests continued, but every time I called them I could sense that things weren't going that smoothly. My results were never great. My hormones weren't multiplying as much as it should. They called me one day at about the seven week mark (just a few days before my first ultrasound, when I'd have the chance to hear the heartbeat of my baby) and said that they'd keep watching my blood test results because it wasn't quite what they were looking for. This wasn't good news. I could sense that things might be going downhill fast and could see the writing on the wall. I remember lying on the spare bed crying and saying to my husband that I could handle two things, but not three. I could do IVF, and I could power through the OHSS, but I couldn't also lose the baby. Losing the baby would break me. It was my tipping point. It would be more than I could handle.

But it wasn't for me to choose because two days before my scheduled ultrasound in January 2014, they said the pregnancy wasn't viable. They told me to go in that afternoon and see the Doctor. I was devastated. My heart felt like it had been ripped from my body and broken into a million pieces. Words can't even describe the devastation I felt. I'd just invested every moment of the last two years of my life, and gone through hell, just to have a miscarriage. Just to have my soul crushed? Once again I was thrust into a deep desperation and confusion, analysing whether there was anything I could have done differently to change this inevitable outcome.

That night, I lay in the spare bed with my swollen stomach and nearly broke Google while I searched for ways this could be wrong. I searched for stories of other women in this situation who turned out ok. Grasped and clutched onto any glimmer of hope that might be out there that I might still be able to carry a healthy baby. I spent hours scouring the internet and came up only with the faintest of hope and an understanding that things were far from ideal.

Lesson 6: Knowledge is power, but trust your medical team

I arrived at the clinic the next day full of questions. It was the same Doctor who'd done my egg retrieval, the one who'd never even said hello to me as he was about to strip my dignity away as I lay, unconscious on the bed, while his instruments punched through my parts and sucked the eggs out of my ovaries. I was disarmed by his kind nature on this occasion and respected his honesty and frank medical opinion. But, how were they sure? What if there was a baby inside that was still alive? I asked the Doctor what felt like a million questions and he made a stunningly obvious point.

"Terminating pregnancies is not our business. This doesn't do our success rates any good," he said. "We wouldn't tell you this news if we weren't sure that this wasn't a viable pregnancy."

He went onto explain that because my progesterone levels were so high, my body wouldn't recognise this and expel the pregnancy for quite some time. I'd be three or four months along by the time I naturally miscarried, and so there was a real chance that the 'mass' (mass? Ahem… baby) would continue to grow larger, at least for another four weeks, by which time the miscarriage would be more painful and more taxing on my body. Not only that, but there'd be a higher chance that I'd be required to come into the hospital for a D&C to have it removed. The alternative was going back for more tests for a week to give me more clarity and confirmation that this was a sad outcome, or wait until it naturally passed. It was at that moment that I truly chose to trust my clinic, my team of specialists and take the recommended course of action, a medical miscarriage. My healthy lifestyle and past medical experiences had left me sceptical and untrusting of the medical industry and I was tired of always second guessing their advice. I needed to reserve my energy and fighting spirit to just surviving each and every day and I didn't want to make that decision. In that moment, I chose trust.

For the first time I fully realised that these people we experts. They were called specialists for a reason. Because they had spent years studying, and then specialising, and then gaining experience and dealing with people, who couldn't successfully conceive, day in and day out for years. Although I had read as much information as I could, there was no comparison for what they knew and had experienced. I had tried to fall pregnant on my own and it hadn't worked and here I was more than two years later, still not pregnant. It was time to put my faith in this team and release the last bits of control, and let them handle the game plan while I worked on how I was going to emotionally survive the most devastating blow of my life.

The only differences between a medical miscarriage and an abortion are intent. Someone who had an abortion didn't want their baby, yet here I was, desperate for one. And whether or not it was a healthy baby. Clearly mine was not. Medically though, they're the same. Two different medications, one to expel the uterine lining and another to induce contractions. As I write this I can still feel the aching in my heart and tears well in my eyes. I had chosen to trust my medical team and accept that this pregnancy would not have a happy ending, but it was like mother nature didn't get to choose. Instead, this pregnancy would end at my own hands. Here I was doing the complete opposite of what I had wanted to two years of my life. I had just invested two years and for what? An abortion? To be brought to my knees with dispair? An indescribable sadness? To this day, I still long for that lost soul and wonder what his or her story would have been.

Without a doubt this was the lowest point in my life.

The medical miscarriage took place at home. Alone. I was warned there would be side effects: hot flushes, nausea, cramps, upset stomach, bleeding, sweating, dizziness, and more. And I had it all. I lay on the bed with a heat pack, some water and strong painkillers as the waves of cramps came over me. They grew stronger and stronger, as I fumbled my way back and forth from the ensuite to throw up and pass clots of blood in a dizzy, foggy haze. I don't know why, but I was desperate to see the foetus and would carefully analyse the blood each time I went to the bathroom. Perhaps it was for closure. The hot flushes became unbearable. The bed sheets were drenched with sweat as I lay there alone in pain and in misery. At one point I thought things seemed terribly wrong. Could you die of a miscarriage? I called the fertility clinic and spoke with one of the nurses who assured me that, unfortunately, these were the normal side effects of the medications, but that if I was still feeling the same at 1.00pm I should call them back. As if my body could tell the time, at 12.30pm on the dot, things finally began to calm down inside me and I was able to rest, physically ok, but emotionally torn.

What followed was a haze of depression. I went to work two days later, pretending nothing had happened. I had become an open book on my journey and felt comfortable with everyone knowing our situation, until now. The two bosses knew because I needed to explain to them why I was missing work. Our parents knew too, but I closed up and shut down and didn't want to have to tell anyone else. All I had wanted to do was cry every moment of every day. I didn't feel like getting out of bed, and I didn't feel like facing the world. I did not know if I could bear another untold story inside me. Was this it for us? We had fully invested two years of our lives (and our finances) into this failed mission. One of the hardest things I had to deal with was my hair falling out in clumps. My hair had always given me a sense of pride. It was unruly, but long and thick and wavy, but now, every shower fully blocked the drain and I'd have to pick up these handfuls of hair every time to throw them out. Every time I brushed my hair, I needed to clean the hairbrush, and my back was full of strands. I lost almost two thirds of my hair by the end. I felt like I had some understanding at that point of how female cancer patients felt when they lose their hair. It is such a physical reminder of how everything has turned to shit.

Yet the questions from friends and family kept coming. I think it was a mix of curiosity and concern. They weren't to know what to say to us or how to act so it wasn't their fault, but I just wished they would stop and I could be left alone. I just didn't want anyone else to try and compare their situation to mine. I knew of people who had gone through miscarriages, but they hadn't spent years trying to have a child or already had one, and they hadn't just had OHSS, and they didn't have to terminate it themselves either, so I didn't want anyone's sympathy or understanding. As far as everyone else was concerned the IVF was unsuccessful and now we were taking a break from fertility treatments.

I had a follow up appointment with my specialist shortly after that. I had dusted myself off a little and stopped wallowing in my own pity by this point. My specialist had asked how I was going, and I went through the motions. "I'm fine. I think I'm handling this all very well actually. It's all part of the process. I can deal with it. Really, I'm fine," I replied. He saw right through me. He looked me square in the eyes and said "No you're not. You're angry." I was taken aback. I had acknowledged my feelings of sadness and depression, but had never stopped to think that I might be angry and I had never expected that to come out of his mouth at all, let alone so directly. "You're angry that it failed. You're angry you got sick and that the pregnancy wasn't viable. You're angry that it is taking so long. You're angry that everywhere you look there are pregnant women and that all your friends are pregnant and having children. You're angry because you're healthy and it's unfair that people who shouldn't be having children can, and you can't," he said matter of factly. For once, I had no words. He was right. All this time, I'd been trying to cover up this intense anger at the world. I wasn't angry at anyone in particular. I didn't feel anger towards my friends when they had children. Sadness, yes, but anger, no. But I was really angry at the world and at the situation and I'd been harbouring this feeling inside me. He was 100% right. I just wanted to scream "F*ck!!! Screw Infertility!"

Lesson 7: You're stronger than you think. You will survive this.

I just wanted to be happy again and live my life. I hadn't taken leave from work in such a long time and I just needed to escape. I needed to stop and repair my tired, broken heart. I needed to start working on getting through this, for real. We made the last minute decision to go overseas for a week to Lombok, a small set of islands in Indonesia, said to be what Bali was like 20 years ago. We stayed at a remote eco-resort that didn't even have hot water (although as if it was needed!) and an eccentric owner who had originated from New Zealand. There were only two other guests at the hotel when we arrived, and only seven (including us) when we left. It was just what we needed. My husband surfed while I read books, had massages, swam in the pool and spoke with the local staff. My hair was still falling out in chunks, a reminder to me that I couldn't truly run away and escape from my problems and I still didn't know what we were going to do, but it felt like the break we needed. And we were forced to recognise how lucky in life we were as we witnessed first-hand the poverty people in third world countries live in. Despite my situation, I began to reflect and truly appreciate the country and situation I had been born into. Returning home though was like a rocket crashing back down to earth. Suddenly we were thrust back into reality.

I have always said to myself that I could be happy without children, but it was the unsuccessful trying that was toughest. In reality, how do you actually take a break from trying to have children? You're either actively trying not to fall pregnant, or you're having unprotected sex and secretly hoping it will take…. Which, really, let's be honest, is trying. I still didn't want to tell anyone, but for some reason, one day I ran into an older friend who didn't have any children and poured my heart out. She confided in me that she had undergone IVF back in the day when you had to lay flat on your back in a hospital bed for two weeks. Her story is for her book, not this one, but as mentioned, children are not part of it. And she is amazing. And confident. And successful. And alive. She survived, and not only did she survive the heartache, the years of trying and the incredible lows, but she was living life. It made me feel like whatever happened, I'd get through it, and finally, I could let out the secret inside me to someone who I connected with. But she looked at me and said "You're not done trying. If you're unsure, then you're not done, and you're still young. Trust your instinct," she said. And so I did.

Becoming vegan had (surprisingly) affected me mentally as well. It is an indescribable feeling of inner peace to stop consuming animal products like nothing I've ever felt before. A well-known vegan, Kris Carr, had written about affirmations in her book, *Crazy Sexy Diet*, but at the time I thought she sounded like a halfwit hippy who lived in la la land. Then I read *Make Peace with your Plate*, by Jess Ainscough (dec), who mentioned that she would repeat to herself 'I truly and deeply love and accept myself' whenever she felt nervous or scared. I also saw the same affirmation in a documentary, and just one day, out of the blue, I got in the shower and started saying it, over and over again.

I said it in the car on the way to and from work.

I said it while I was walking around the office.

I said it in front of the mirror.

The first time I said it, I thought I sounded like an idiot. I didn't love and accept myself - life was crap and I hated it and I was angry at the world. It was like I was just trying to convince myself of something I didn't believe, but I kept going. I had nothing to lose, and nowhere to go but up, and, each time I said it, it got easier. Each time I said it, I believed it a little bit more. I had started shifting the energy in my body from the heavy burden of what we were going through, to reminding myself, constantly, to show myself love and that I would pull out of this struggle.

Lesson 8: Be your biggest cheerleader

I became my biggest cheerleader. The best thing about being your own cheerleader, is that nobody else has to know about it - you can cheer yourself on, tell yourself that everything is going to be ok, constantly, and you can do it all in your head. I kept saying my affirmations and really focusing on changing my outlook and literally one day I just woke up and felt in myself that I could handle anything anyone threw at me. Just like that. I was prepared to do just about anything to have this baby, and I could do this. Hell no, I really wasn't ready to give up yet! It didn't mean that I thought I'd coast through things and that it would be a piece of cake. It didn't mean that all of a sudden I wasn't angry. It didn't mean that I'd forgotten the sadness of the little person that may have been growing inside me. The truth is that I can still feel all those feelings in my soul but they're not as intense as they were before, and more importantly, I could cope. I'd developed grit and resilience. That ability to accept and absorb the failure and the lows, and not let them debilitate me. That ability to fall and dust myself off and then get back up again. And the ability to recognise my feelings, acknowledge and accept them, and move on with life. I was becoming a survivor.

We returned to the clinic. I had since had a test that showed there might be something wrong with me - my immune system was switched on, big time. Was it rheumatoid arthritis? Lupus? It could have been one of about 100 things, but in that moment, all I could think of was that I might be the cause of our infertility. There was an arrogance about me that thought that all along this surely couldn't have been my doing. I was healthy. I had taken every possible measure to try and make this happen. I was seeing a naturopath. I was militant about my diet and I was taking a host of supplements. Surely I wasn't the missing link? But then I was. Or could be. My husband and I have always tried to be a team, and made a vow to never argue about whose fault it was, but when the finger is pointed at you, it hurts. And then a million and one other thoughts raced through my mind. All this time wasted and d the drain because of a simple test. Had they done this test previously? What would happen if I had one of these diseases? Had my body attacked the embryo and killed it when I'd had the miscarriage? Had I done something to cause this? Despite running a number of tests, we never found out the cause of it, and I was put on cortico-steroids, the same medication as some cancer patients, to treat whatever might be there, as well as aspirin. In combination, the plan was to surpress my immune system to prevent it from attacking any foreign bodies... like babies. I had been humbled by those test results, and put back in my place, even if I had tried to bury my past feelings, and left in awe of just how many things could be uncovered on this journey. I really needed to trust my medical team.

In April we tried once more with two the frozen embryos. That was all we had left. I recalled a previous conversation with our specialist when I was lectured about the risks with twins and triplets and how we really didn't want that to occur. I remember nodding while at the same time crossing my toes and secretly hoping that we could just fall pregnant with twins so that this would all be over, completely ignoring what he said. This time though, the specialist had suggested putting both of the eggs back in, not us. Was it a sign that he was beginning to get desperate? Was it a sign that he didn't have much confidence in those eggs? Most probably the latter, as we discovered that the embryos still had never really multiplied much. But we were hopeful. As this was an FET (Frozen Embryo Transfer) the drug protocol was so much easier, despite my new regime of 'immune system killer drugs'. This time around felt different though. My attitude had changed. I had changed. I was saying my affirmations all the time and writing in my gratitude journal, and even rubbing my belly and willing it to be pregnant, visualising myself as a gorgeous pregnant goddess and picturing myself as a mother. But it wasn't so much that I felt so much more confident. It was that I felt I was stronger now and could handle the failure and all of the kinks and turns that may have been to come. I felt like a warrior. We waited nervously once again, only to discover that as usual, the result was negative. Disappointing as usual, but not soul crushing as it had been on previous occasions.

Once again, we found ourselves at the fertility clinic, ready to find out what the next step would be and nervous as hell that history would repeat itself. So then we reached the peak of fertility treatments – ICSI. Because we were able to retrieve a lot of eggs, but not many fertilised, they were now going to do the fertilisation for us. Mother nature was now sitting on the couch watching Netflix while science took over. I was concerned that I'd suffer complications again, but my specialist assured me that things would be different this time around. With the exception of my daily drugs to combat my immune system going haywire, all my drugs were changed (again), and they managed my hormones in a different way. How many drugs and how many different treatments were there? The science behind it blew my mind. I felt like they were keeping a much closer eye on me this time around, but my body still went to work, producing an incredible number of eggs. At one ultrasound they counted 46.

The time had come for the retrieval again. The last one felt like a fun excursion to a luxury hotel (minus a few things here and there, but you know), except this time I was informed that the private hospital was full and I'd have to have my day surgery in the public hospital. This isn't what I signed up for. I felt like a snob, but I'd paid top dollar for my private hotel room health cover. I'd been going through hell and back, and got dumped in a room with another 20 people, no TV, no magazines and my husband couldn't even come in with me. I sobbed, feeling sorry for myself (It's my pity party and I'll cry if I want to) as I waited until I was pulled into surgery. As they wheeled me in, I discovered that I had the same specialist doing my retrieval, and like Groundhog Day, there he was, sitting at his computer, not even bothered about saying hello. Whatever, I knew the drill. The surgery was much like the previous one, and they had extracted 19 eggs. But after the surgery I was in agonising pain. One of the nurses from the clinic came to tell me how many eggs they'd retrieved and I was doubled over in pain, in my public hospital corridor. A lovely nurse came over and upped my pain relief. My body wasn't absorbing my drip very quickly either but she kept checking on me and helping me with more pain relief. This was different to the last time. I was in so much pain, and I felt awfully dizzy and weak. They brought me over some sandwiches and I managed to eat a quarter. I just felt too ill. So I lay there, falling in and out of sleep.

Then, the shift changed. A new nurse was looking after me, and she wanted me out. I was no longer a person, I was a bed that needed to be made available. She grabbed the intravenous liquid bag and squeezed it to make the liquid enter my body faster, and then told me to make my way to the bathroom and get changed because I was being discharged. I asked for help to walk and put on my shoes, but I waited 15 minutes and nobody came. I slowly shuffled, edging my way to the bathroom, and returned and wrestled with my shoes for another five minutes, before she conveniently returned and said in a sarcastically surprised tone "oh, you could do it yourself?" My husband wasn't even allowed to come in and get me, so I had to shuffle out slowly on my own to find him, as it felt like someone had punched me hard from the inside of my stomach. As we started walking to the car, I collapsed. I just wasn't well. I sat on the pavement outside the hospital while he got the car, and helped me get into it. I was no better when we arrived home either. He carried me inside and lay me on the bed and helped me undress, and then got me a heat bag and some painkillers. My body was exhausted and sore, and then as I lay there, I felt an incredible surge of pain rip through my shoulder. I couldn't move. I was paralysed, and I wailed for Ross as loudly as I could, but he had walked outside for a brief moment. "Roosssssss", I shrieked, but he didn't come. I was in desperate agony. I just knew I needed to get up, and so I summoned every ounce of my energy and staggered to the dresser and leant up against it, desperately hoping this incredible, sharp pain would pass, and eventually it did. Most likely, a bubble of air from the surgery had made it's way up to my shoulder.

As per usual, the following day, I was sore but able, and as the retrievals are almost always held on a Friday, I had the weekend to recover. My retrieval was on Monday though, so it would be one more day before I returned to work. I had heard many stories and knew many people who would just leave work for their transfer and then return afterwards, but I was done being a hero. I was all about looking after me now. As we prepared for our transfer, the doctor looked at me, squeezed my shoulder and said "oh honey, you've had a rough trot, haven't you?" All I could think was "Oh god, they all know me!" The results this time were much more encouraging though. Of the 14 eggs they thought were suitable, 10 had fertilised, one was ready for transfer, and five had made it to the freezer. Just like the last cycle, I was now an emotional warrior. Physically, there was no sign of OHSS and I had recovered from the surgery. When I decided that I would continue with fertility treatments, I had decided that I was all in. I would wait until the specialist had lost all hope or the finances ran out or until I just knew that I couldn't do it anymore. I was prepared for failure. But I was planning for success.

Just like the last cycle, I was secretly cheering myself on inside. It's so empowering to be your biggest cheerleader. And what we don't realise too, is that all of the most successful people in the world are their biggest cheerleaders too. Elite athlete type who go to the Olympics - all have psychologists who recommend all of these things to them. They make sure their body is in peak physical shape, they test all the different scenarios, and they are constantly visualising a gold medal. They are constantly picturing themselves on a podium, singing the national anthem of their country. They're visualising themselves with their hands in the air shouting "yes!" They're always telling themselves they can do it. When they break a bone, they don't give up, they focus on recovery and then they get straight back up and try again. They meditate. They show gratitude. They're warriors.

And I'd become a warrior too. And I still am. I constantly visualised myself pregnant, and had this vision of myself walking down the street holding hands with a little girl. I said affirmations constantly. I looked after myself - when I wanted to rest, I did, and if I didn't want to see my friends, I didn't. And I looked after my body too.

And once again I fell pregnant. I'm not saying that positive psychology helped me fall pregnant, although studies have shown that the odds of success with fertility treatments are greatly increased, even doubled, with the use of mind body techniques like relaxation and meditation, and positive psychology. I don't think anyone can guarantee that you'll fall pregnant. It isn't a given, but these are skills that last us a lifetime and help us in so many scenarios, beyond this rollercoaster of infertility.

Given our previous scenario, I knew there was a real chance of miscarriage again, and I enjoyed having my little secret, because we had still duped everyone except our parents into thinking we were taking a break. At this point in time, I was also enjoying not having to listen to the uneducated comments of other people, and the (unintentional) insensitivity. I had breakfast with some of my girlfriends when I was five weeks along, and one of them asked me "If I had finished grieving yet?" I will never stop grieving the untold story inside me, and especially I feel, because of my situation and the circumstances surrounding the loss. "And I've spoken with Andrew and agreed that if you need a surrogate then we'd do that for you," she said. I could appreciate the sentiment, but was stunned at the naivety of the comment, and speechless. I didn't have a problem (as far as I knew) with carrying a child. I didn't need a surrogate. As quickly as she had blurted it out, I changed the topic, and resolved to keep my secret a little longer.

Lesson 9: Everyone just wants the best for you. Understand that despite all their questions, prying and misguided advice, deep down, they're really hoping you fall pregnant too.

At 14 weeks pregnant though, the time had come for me to begin looking for a replacement at work, and so we let the cat out of the bag to our extended family, friends and work colleagues. I'll never forget the joy people felt as we told them the news. You don't realise it at the time, but when you tell people about your infertility, even though it might not feel like it, these people want you to fall pregnant too. These people are hoping and praying that you'll have a baby, and are on your journey with you. And when you fall pregnant, they feel it too. They share in your highs, and feel your relief, your joy and your happiness.

Some people get irritated when others feel their pregnant belly. I was delighted every time, because I felt like it was rubbing a Buddha for good luck. I always felt like I'd never have the chance to have the chance for people to rub my belly! Still, there was a part of me that, at every appointment prepared for bad news. Emotionally I could cope, but I just couldn't believe that it was happening. It was surreal. I had a wonderful pregnancy, and I was very zen about everything. I decided that I would 'go with the flow' and put my complete and utter trust in my medical team, and focus on my emotional and physical wellness. During my fertility journey I surrendered and released control, to focus on keeping myself well and it had worked. I would do the same this time around.

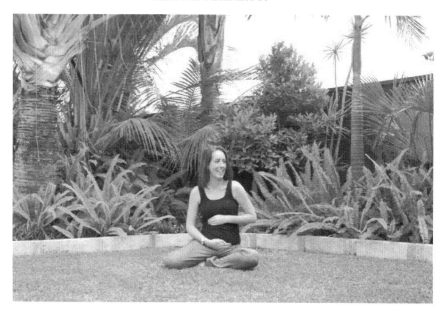

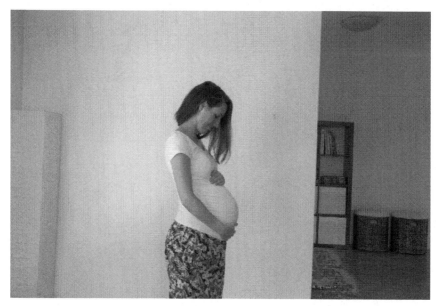

Lesson 10: Baby or not, at some point, the marathon will end.

I went into labour about four days before my due date, and things went a little pear-shaped while she was making her way into the world, but when we saw Chloe's face, Ross and I both burst into tears. In an instant, the dark clouds that had been weighing us down had lifted.

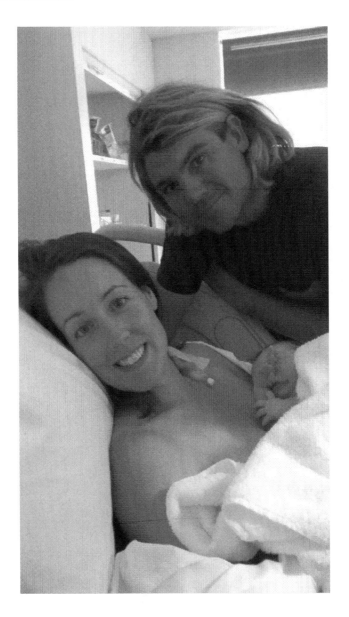

We had done it. Finally. Will everyone in this situation fall pregnant? The honest answer is no, and the odds are stacked against us. Each day there are more and more chemicals surrounding us, the air becomes more polluted, and our diets are on a downward spiral while we wait until we're older to begin families. The success rates for IVF (in-vitro fertilisation) are still less than 50%.

My journey is one of success. I would never wish this experience on anyone else but for better or worse, I'm a changed person. A warrior.

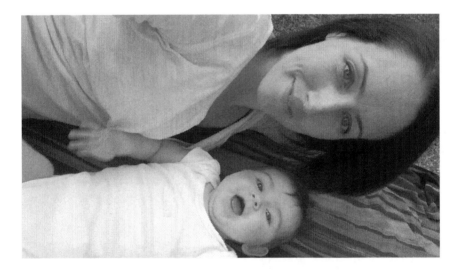

For Ross and I, this roller coaster will reignite soon as we begin treatments once again for a second child. On the surface I feel like it will be easier, although friends who have walked in these shoes tell me it's the same highs and lows all over again.

But for now....

I've always compared infertility to a marathon. I'd prepared for a 100m sprint, and ended up running a marathon. I didn't know where the finish line was, and there were hurdles everywhere, and I felt like finally I got to stop jogging.

I decided to write this book because I never want women with infertility to feel as low as I felt.

I was sick of people telling me not to stress and then not providing me with strategies to cope with my stress, and I wanted to provide an honest and raw account of my experience to help friends and family trying to help a loved one with infertility.

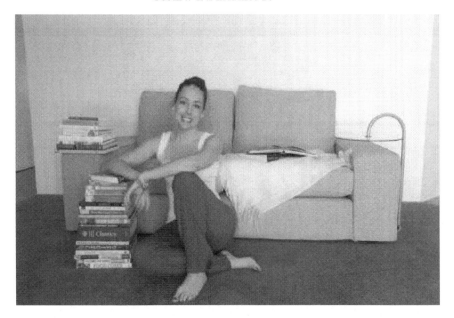

About the Author

Robyn Birkin is a blogger, fertility warrior and zen mama who lives in Perth, Western Australia with her husband and daughter, Chloe, a gorgeous result of IVF treatments.

After getting married and travelling the world, at the age of 30, Robyn and her husband decided to start a family, but after 12 heartbreaking months of trying alone, finally accepted that they had infertility. What came next was a gruelling year and a half of invasive fertility treatments, complications from medications and a soul crushing miscarriage.

On her quest to fall pregnant and manage the incredible stress caused by treatments, Robyn researched, asked questions and reached out to others, discovering a number of powerful strategies to not only help her survive infertility, but thrive despite it.

In this book, Robyn reveals her heartfelt, moving and inspiring journey, and uses her experience to share the lessons she learnt on this life changing journey from trying to conceive to motherhood.

You can find Robyn here:

Website: http://moderndaymissus.com
Facebook: https://www.facebook.com/moderndaymissus
Instagram: http://instagram.com/moderndaymissus
Twitter: https://twitter.com/moderndaymissus

Private Fertility Warriors Facebook Support + Chat Group
A safe and welcoming place to feel vulnerable
A place to vent when nobody else around you understands what you're going through
A forum to ask questions you can't ask your Doctor
A place to learn hints and tips from people who know and understand

https://facebook.com/groups/fertilitywarriors

Made in the USA
Lexington, KY
14 August 2019